day one

Meal	Ingredients	Calories	Proteins (g)	Fats (g)	Carbs (g)	Therm X Max Cut Pro
Breakfast	Scrambled eggs with vegetables	300	20	18	10	1 capsule
Snack	Greek yogurt with berries	150	10	2	25	-
Lunch	Grilled chicken breast with mixed greens and balsamic dressing	400	30	12	35	-
Snack	Apple slices with almond butter	200	3	15	20	-
Dinner	Baked salmon with roasted vegetables	450	35	20	30	-
Therm X Max Cut Pro	1 capsule with lunch	-	-	-	-	-
Total		1500	98	67	120	-

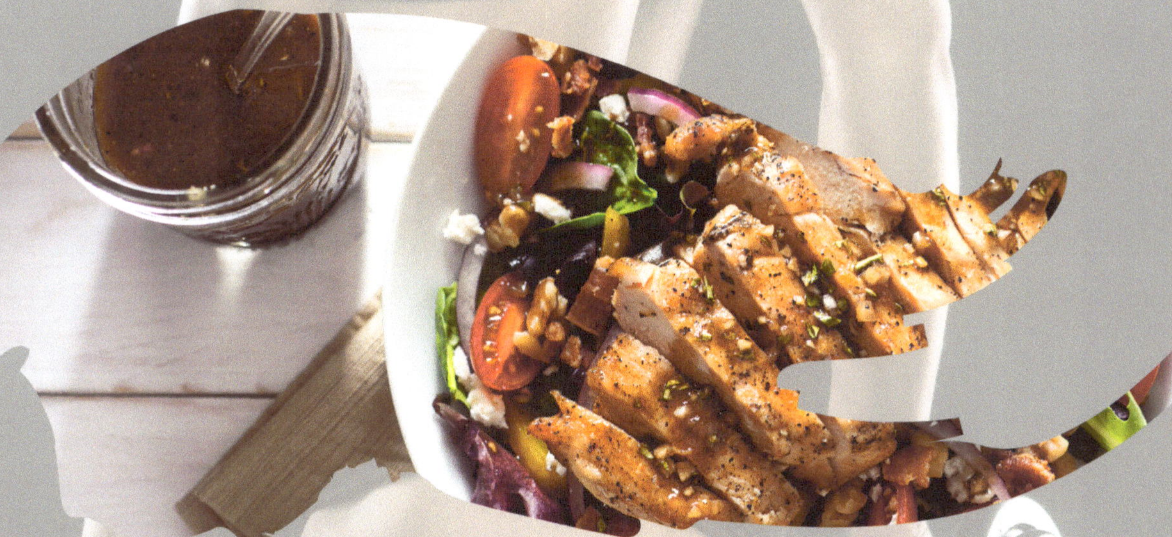

Remember to drink plenty of water throughout the day and adjust portion sizes and meal components based on your specific dietary needs and preferences. This is a general guide and may not be suitable for everyone. Always consult with a healthcare provider before starting any new diet or supplement regimen.

Please note that the use of the Therm X Max Cut Pro supplement should be started with 1 capsule in the morning to assess your tolerance. If well-tolerated, you may then move to 2 capsules per day, as suggested earlier.

the levi method

date

your mood

water tracker

today's big goal

notes

schedule

6:00

7:00

8:00

9:00

10:00

11:00

12:00

13:00

14:00

15:00

16:00

17:00

18:00

19:00

20:00

21:00

day one minute by minute

7:00 AM	Wake up, hydrate with a glass of water
7:30 AM	Breakfast: Scrambled eggs on whole grain toast Calories: 300 Protein: 20g Carbs: 30g Fat: 12g
7:45 AM	Take 1-2 capsules of Therm X Max Cut Pro with a glass of water
10:00 AM	Snack: Apple Calories: 80 Protein: 0g Carbs: 20g Fat: 0g
12:30 PM	Lunch: Grilled chicken salad with olive oil dressing Calories: 400 Protein: 35g Carbs: 10g Fat: 25g
3:00 PM	Snack: Greek yogurt with mixed berries Calories: 150 Protein: 12g Carbs: 18g Fat: 3g
4:00 PM	25-minute light walk
6:30 PM	Dinner: Grilled salmon with quinoa and steamed vegetables Calories: 600 Protein: 40g Carbs: 50g Fat: 25g
8:00 PM	Snack: A handful of almonds Calories: 160 Protein: 6g Carbs: 6g Fat: 14g
10:00 PM	Rest and recovery for the next day

something to think about...

When it comes to weight loss, the perspective you adopt towards your goals can make all the difference. Rather than setting a daunting target of losing 5 kilograms, consider reframing your goal: **aim to lose 1 kilogram, five times.**

Breaking down your weight loss journey into manageable increments makes the process seem less **intimidating and more achievable**. This way, you're not staring at a distant finish line, but instead focusing on a series of smaller, attainable goals. Each kilogram lost becomes a victory, a sign of progress, and a boost to your motivation.

Think of each kilogram as a stepping-stone on your path to weight loss. As you reach each milestone, take a moment to celebrate your success. Rewarding yourself can have a profound impact on your motivation, encouraging you to continue moving forward.

Moreover, this perspective shift allows for better tracking of your progress. Instead of waiting to celebrate until you've lost the full 5 kilograms, you get to enjoy five distinct moments of achievement. This not only keeps you motivated but also provides constant feedback on your efforts, enabling you to adjust your approach if needed.

Remember, weight loss is not a race; it's a journey. And on this journey, every kilogram lost is a win worth celebrating. Adopting this mindset can turn what once felt like a marathon into a series of satisfying sprints. So, aim for losing 1 kilogram, five times, and witness how this shift in perspective can revolutionize your weight loss journey.

the levi method

date

your mood

water tracker

today´s big goal

notes

schedule

6:00

7:00

8:00

9:00

10:00

11:00

12:00

13:00

14:00

15:00

16:00

17:00

18:00

19:00

20:00

21:00

day two

Meal	Ingredients	Calories	Proteins (g)	Fats (g)	Carbs (g)	Therm X Max Cut Pro
Breakfast	Oatmeal with sliced bananas	300	10	5	55	1 capsule
Snack	Carrot sticks with hummus	100	2	6	10	-
Lunch	Beef stir-fry with broccoli and brown rice	450	25	15	50	-
Snack	Oreo Grenade bar	250	4	12	35	-
Dinner	Grilled pork tenderloin with roasted sweet potatoes	500	30	20	40	-
Therm X Max Cut Pro	1 capsule with breakfast	-	-	-	-	-
Total		1600	71	58	190	-

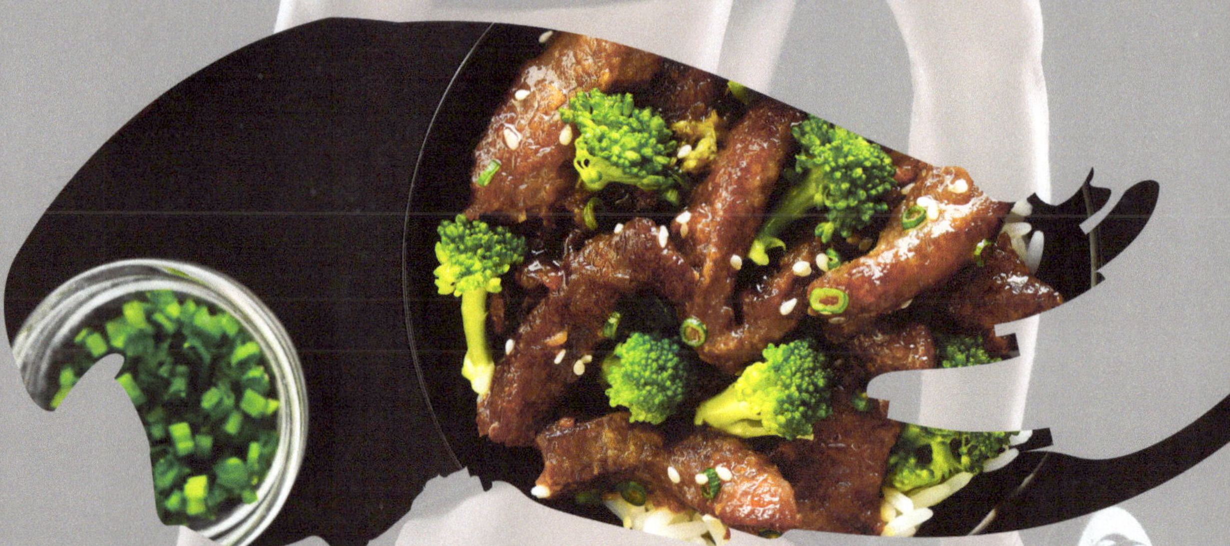

Remember to drink plenty of water throughout the day and adjust portion sizes and meal components based on your specific dietary needs and preferences. This is a general guide and may not be suitable for everyone. Always consult with a healthcare provider before starting any new diet or supplement regimen.

Please note that the use of the Therm X Max Cut Pro supplement should be started with 1 capsule in the morning to assess your tolerance. If well-tolerated, you may then move to 2 capsules per day, as suggested earlier.

the levi method

date

schedule

your mood

6:00

7:00

8:00

water tracker

9:00

10:00

today's big goal

11:00

12:00

13:00

notes

14:00

15:00

16:00

17:00

18:00

19:00

20:00

21:00

the science behind it_

Okay, cool peeps! So you've decided to lose a few pounds, correct? You're probably wondering where to begin and how all of this weight loss nonsense works. So, how about we break it down?

The 'Caloric Deficit' is the main attraction on our weight loss show. Doesn't that sound fancy? It certainly isn't! The term 'caloric deficit' simply means 'eat less, move more.' Simple as that.

Let's start with the food. Food serves as fuel for your body. It keeps your engine running and gives you the energy you need to get through the day. Every time you eat that delicious burger or drink that super thick milkshake, your body says, "Cool, let's store this energy for later!" But here's the thing: if you keep storing energy and not using it, it will turn into fat. To lose weight, you must consume fewer calories than your body requires to maintain its current weight. And how do we go about doing so? You've got to cut back on your energy consumption, pal! This does not imply that you must forego food. Simply make healthier choices, such as replacing that milkshake with a fruity smoothie.

Let's move on to the second part: moving more. Physical activity is similar to a calorie-burning party. When you dance to your favourite song or go for a run, your body says, "Alright, let's burn some of that stored energy!" The more you move, the more calories you burn, and the easier it is to maintain your caloric deficit. It's like throwing a party where the uninvited guests are the calories you're trying to sneak out!

And here's the best part: combining the two - eating less and moving more - is a one-two punch to those extra pounds! By doing both, you're addressing the caloric deficit from both sides, making it easier and faster to meet your weight loss goals. But keep in mind that you must be consistent. This isn't a one-time occurrence. It's a way of life shift.

Remember, it's not about being skinny or looking like the magazine cover models. It's all about feeling good about yourself and staying healthy. So be gentle with your body. It will return the favour if you treat it well. Cheers to starting your weight loss journey with the caloric deficit! Let's do it, friends!

day three

Meal	Ingredients	Calories	Proteins (g)	Fats (g)	Carbs (g)	Therm X Max Cut Pro
Breakfast	Vegetable omelette	350	20	25	10	1 capsule
Snack	Cottage cheese with pineapple chunks	150	15	2	20	-
Lunch	Grilled chicken salad with mixed greens and lemon vinaigrette	400	30	18	25	-
Snack	Celery sticks with peanut butter	200	5	16	10	-
Dinner	Beef and vegetable stir-fry with quinoa	450	25	15	45	-
Therm X Max Cut Pro	1 capsule with dinner	-	-	-	-	-
Total		1550	95	76	110	-

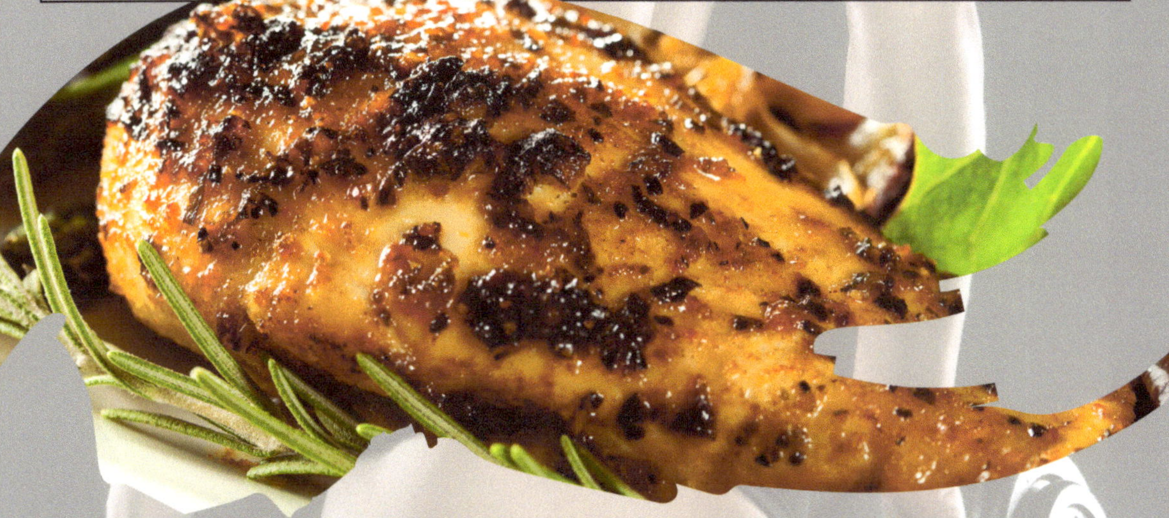

Remember to drink plenty of water throughout the day and adjust portion sizes and meal components based on your specific dietary needs and preferences. This is a general guide and may not be suitable for everyone. Always consult with a healthcare provider before starting any new diet or supplement regimen.

Please note that the use of the Therm X Max Cut Pro supplement should be started with 1 capsule in the morning to assess your tolerance. If well-tolerated, you may then move to 2 capsules per day, as suggested earlier.

the levi method

date

your mood

water tracker

today's big goal

notes

schedule

6:00

7:00

8:00

9:00

10:00

11:00

12:00

13:00

14:00

15:00

16:00

17:00

18:00

19:00

20:00

21:00

this is neat_

You ready to dive deeper into this calorie-burning business? Let's talk about Total Daily Energy Expenditure, or TDEE as the cool kids call it.
So, your TDEE is like the total amount of energy you burn in a day, the ultimate calorie incinerator.

But it's not just one big thing. It's like a super team of four calorie-busting heroes. Let's meet 'em, shall we?
First up, we have our Basal Metabolic Rate (BMR) - the silent hero. This is the amount of energy your body needs to just exist, like running your heart, lungs, and brain when you're binge-watching your favorite show. It's your body's base energy needs, hence the 'basal' part.

Then we have the Thermic Effect of Food (TEF). Think of this as the energy cost of eating. I know, right? Eating burns calories! Who knew? Well, your body uses energy to digest, absorb, and store the food you eat. So, next time you're munching on an apple, remember you're burning some calories too!

Next up, we have Non-Exercise Activity Thermogenesis (NEAT). Now, this is all the energy you burn by just doing your everyday stuff, like walking your dog, playing air guitar, or even fidgeting during a boring class. So, don't underestimate the power of daily movements.
Last, but definitely not least, is Exercise Activity Thermogenesis (EAT). This one's pretty straightforward. It's all the energy you burn through deliberate exercise, like jogging, dancing, or playing soccer with your buddies.

Put these four heroes together, and you get your TDEE, the total amount of calories you burn in a day. The higher your TDEE, the more calories you burn, and the easier it is to create that caloric deficit we talked about. But remember, everyone's TDEE is different. Your body is unique, so what works for your friend may not work for you. Listen to your body and find what feels good for you.

So, there you go! A crash course on TDEE and its super team. Now, go conquer those calories with your newfound knowledge! You've got this, champ!

the levi method

day four

Meal	Ingredients	Calories	Proteins (g)	Fats (g)	Carbs (g)	Therm X Max Cut Pro
Breakfast	Protein smoothie with almond milk, banana, and spinach	350	20	10	45	1 capsule
Snack	Hard-boiled eggs	140	12	10	1	-
Lunch	Pork tenderloin with steamed broccoli and quinoa	450	30	15	40	-
Snack	Oreo Grenade bar	250	4	12	35	-
Dinner	Grilled chicken breast with roasted vegetables and couscous	500	30	12	55	-
Therm X Max Cut Pro	1 capsule with breakfast	-	-	-	-	-
Total		1690	96	59	176	-

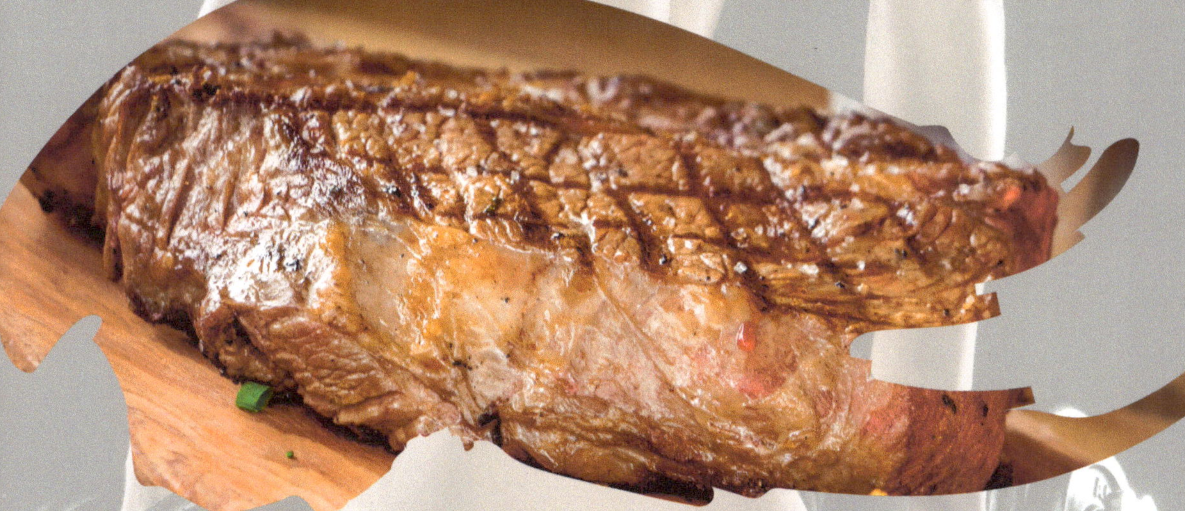

Remember to drink plenty of water throughout the day and adjust portion sizes and meal components based on your specific dietary needs and preferences. This is a general guide and may not be suitable for everyone. Always consult with a healthcare provider before starting any new diet or supplement regimen.

Please note that the use of the Therm X Max Cut Pro supplement should be started with 1 capsule in the morning to assess your tolerance. If well-tolerated, you may then move to 2 capsules per day, as suggested earlier.

the levi method

date

your mood

water tracker

today's big goal

notes

schedule

6:00

7:00

8:00

9:00

10:00

11:00

12:00

13:00

14:00

15:00

16:00

17:00

18:00

19:00

20:00

21:00

day five

Meal	Ingredients	Calories	Proteins (g)	Fats (g)	Carbs (g)	Therm X Max Cut Pro
Breakfast	Vegetable frittata	350	20	25	10	1 capsule
Snack	Greek yogurt with sliced almonds	200	12	10	15	-
Lunch	Beef and vegetable kebabs with brown rice	450	25	18	40	-
Snack	Carrot and cucumber slices with hummus	100	3	5	15	-
Dinner	Grilled pork chops with grilled zucchini and sweet potato	500	30	22	40	-
Therm X Max Cut Pro	1 capsule with lunch	-	-	-	-	-
Total		1600	90	80	120	

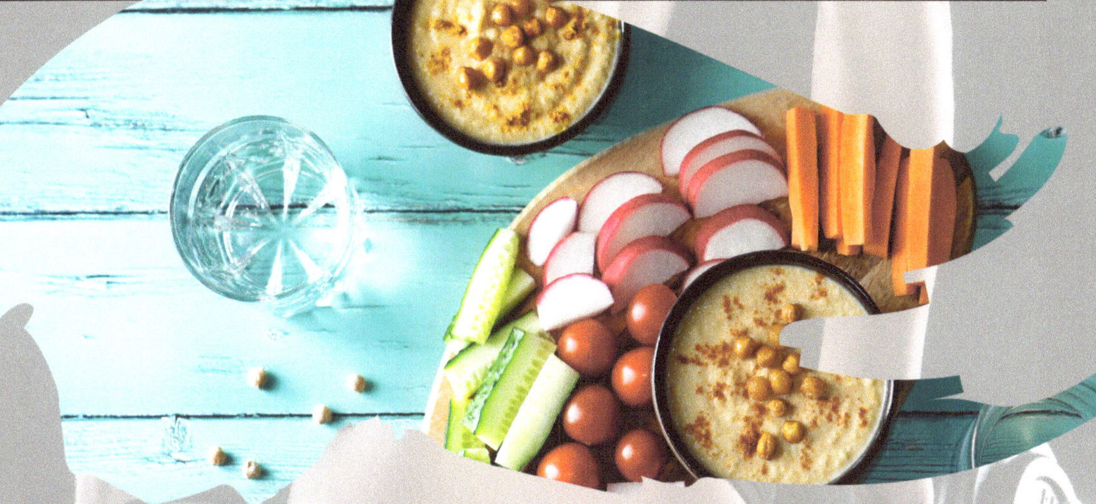

Remember to drink plenty of water throughout the day and adjust portion sizes and meal components based on your specific dietary needs and preferences. This is a general guide and may not be suitable for everyone. Always consult with a healthcare provider before starting any new diet or supplement regimen.

Please note that the use of the Therm X Max Cut Pro supplement should be started with 1 capsule in the morning to assess your tolerance. If well-tolerated, you may then move to 2 capsules per day, as suggested earlier.

the levi method

date

your mood

water tracker

today's big goal

notes

schedule

6:00

7:00

8:00

9:00

10:00

11:00

12:00

13:00

14:00

15:00

16:00

17:00

18:00

19:00

20:00

21:00

training & fat loss:

it's time for us to clear up a little misunderstanding. A lot of folks think the main reason to hit the gym is to burn off those fries from lunch. But let me let you in on a little secret – that's not the whole picture.

When we talk about exercise, we aren't just talking about torching calories. We're talking about leveling up your strength and growing those muscles. Like turning your body into your own personal superhero, right? It's like leveling up in a video game. The more you exercise, the stronger your avatar... err, your body becomes. And who doesn't want to be stronger, right?

Now, don't get it twisted. You still want to burn more calories than you take in if you're looking to drop some fat. But that's mostly gonna come from what you eat, not how many miles you run. Your diet is like your game plan. It's what's gonna guide your progress and help you reach your goals.

So, where does exercise fit in? Well, even though diet is the key player in losing fat, exercise has a pretty sweet side gig. It helps to maintain your muscle mass while you're losing fat. That's like being able to keep all your cool gear while still losing the extra baggage in a game. Pretty rad, right?

But there's more! Exercise also helps to improve your overall body composition. That's a fancy way of saying it changes what your body is made of. Less fat, more muscle – kind of like upgrading your character's armor.

And if that's not enough, exercise also gives your metabolism a boost. That's like getting a speed upgrade in your game. The faster your metabolism, the quicker your body burns through calories.

So, remember guys, exercise isn't just about burning off that extra slice of pizza. It's about building a stronger, more efficient body. And with a well-balanced diet and regular exercise, you can level up your health and fitness game like a champ!

day six

Meal	Ingredients	Calories	Proteins (g)	Fats (g)	Carbs (g)	Therm X Max Cut Pro
Breakfast	Overnight oats with berries and almond milk	350	12	8	60	1 capsule
Snack	Cottage cheese with sliced peaches	150	12	2	20	-
Lunch	Grilled chicken Caesar salad	400	30	20	15	-
Snack	Apple slices with peanut butter	200	5	15	20	-
Dinner	Beef and vegetable stir-fry with cauliflower rice	450	25	15	40	-
Therm X Max Cut Pro	1 capsule with dinner	-	-	-	-	-
Total		1550	84	60	155	-

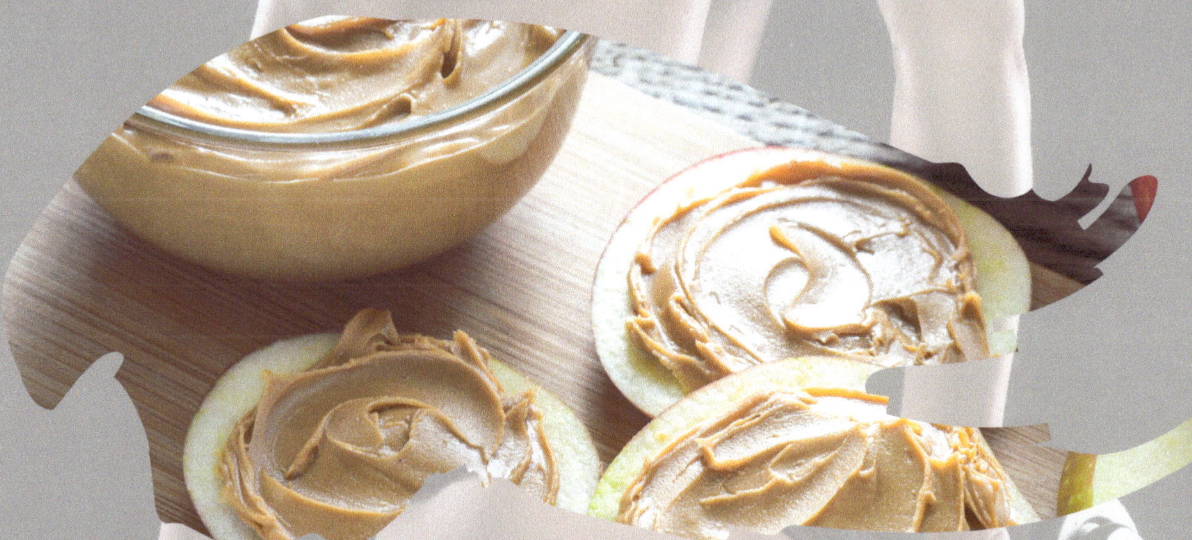

Remember to drink plenty of water throughout the day and adjust portion sizes and meal components based on your specific dietary needs and preferences. This is a general guide and may not be suitable for everyone. Always consult with a healthcare provider before starting any new diet or supplement regimen.

Please note that the use of the Therm X Max Cut Pro supplement should be started with 1 capsule in the morning to assess your tolerance. If well-tolerated, you may then move to 2 capsules per day, as suggested earlier.

the levi method

date

your mood

water tracker

today's big goal

notes

schedule

6:00

7:00

8:00

9:00

10:00

11:00

12:00

13:00

14:00

15:00

16:00

17:00

18:00

19:00

20:00

21:00

tracking progress

Let's take a look at another exciting aspect of your fitness journey. It's similar to getting a high score in a video game, except the game is your health and well-being. We're discussing progress tracking. This may appear to be extra work, but believe me when I say it is a game changer.

The first thing you should know is that progress does not always appear on the scale. Sure, seeing your weight fall can be very satisfying. It's like seeing your game score rise. But keep in mind that the number on the scale can jiggle around like a pinball. It can be influenced by a variety of factors, such as how much water you're drinking, what you ate for dinner last night, or even if you're simply feeling bloated.

That's why we have some other useful tools in our toolbox. Taking body measurements is one of them. Tracking your body's changes with a tape measure can be extremely beneficial. It's similar to receiving a detailed map of your character's journey, showing you exactly where you've made the most progress.

Progress photos are another tool in your arsenal. Consider this your fitness journey's photo album. It serves as a visual reminder of how far you've come and can be extremely motivating. Plus, it's like your own personal before-and-after reveal, and who doesn't love that?

Finally, don't overlook your strength gains in the gym. Remember how we discussed how exercise is all about building strength and muscle? Tracking how much you can lift or how many reps you can do is a great way to see how far you've come. It's like seeing your character's power level increase. Isn't that cool?

So, remember this, my amazing crew: the scale does not tell the whole story. There are numerous methods for tracking your progress and determining how far you've come. Use all of your resources and celebrate every victory, big or small. You're killing it in this game, and I can't wait to see where it takes you!

the levi method

date

your mood

water tracker

today's big goal

notes

schedule

6:00

7:00

8:00

9:00

10:00

11:00

12:00

13:00

14:00

15:00

16:00

17:00

18:00

19:00

20:00

21:00

day seven

Meal	Ingredients	Calories	Proteins (g)	Fats (g)	Carbs (g)	Therm X Max Cut Pro
Breakfast	Scrambled eggs with spinach and bell peppers	300	20	15	10	1 capsule
Snack	Hard-boiled eggs	140	12	10	1	-
Lunch	Grilled pork tenderloin with roasted Brussels sprouts	450	30	20	30	-
Snack	Oreo Grenade bar	250	4	12	35	-
Dinner	Baked chicken breast with roasted asparagus and quinoa	500	30	15	45	-
Therm X Max Cut Pro	1 capsule with breakfast	-	-	-	-	-
Total		1640	96	72	121	-

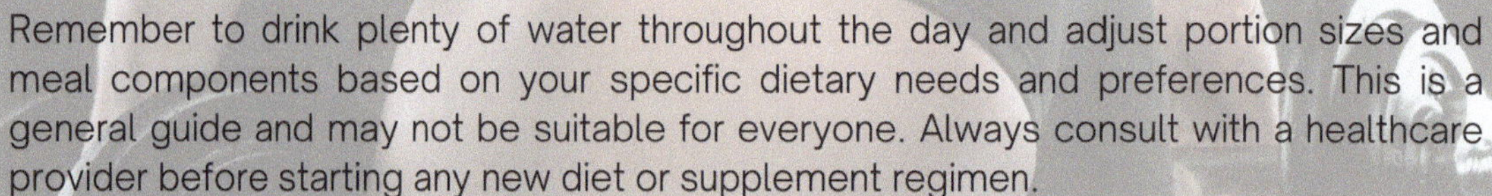

Remember to drink plenty of water throughout the day and adjust portion sizes and meal components based on your specific dietary needs and preferences. This is a general guide and may not be suitable for everyone. Always consult with a healthcare provider before starting any new diet or supplement regimen.

Please note that the use of the Therm X Max Cut Pro supplement should be started with 1 capsule in the morning to assess your tolerance. If well-tolerated, you may then move to 2 capsules per day, as suggested earlier.

the levi method

date

your mood

water tracker

today's big goal

notes

schedule

6:00

7:00

8:00

9:00

10:00

11:00

12:00

13:00

14:00

15:00

16:00

17:00

18:00

19:00

20:00

21:00

the levi method